Self-help
Fibromyalgia

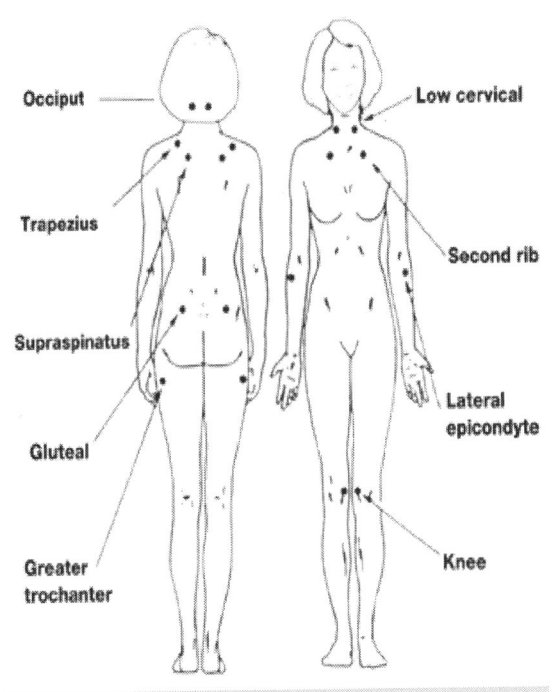

Fibromyalgia diagnostic 'Tender spots'

"Your body will heal itself!"

Angela Bea
SRN, MAR.

Contents.

Introduction Disclaimer

Chapter 1 Illness and Dis-ease

Chapter 2 What do we mean by Fibromyalgia, ME, and CFS? [Fibromyalgia symptoms]

Chapter 3 Dehydration, cell health, acidity and alkalinity

Chapter 4 Good food. Foods to avoid. Basic nutritional facts

Chapter 5 What can I eat and drink? Getting specific

Chapter 6 Therapies and self-help treatments

Chapter 7 How to make life easier

Appendix 1 List of alkaline/acid foods

Appendix 2 Useful books, references and websites

Introduction.

This is intended to be a small self-help book for people and their carers who have been diagnosed with Fibromyalgia, and may also be helpful for those with similar conditions of Chronic Fatigue and ME.

The book is in no way a definitive explanation or medical tome of which there are now many on these conditions. It does not mean to be prescriptive or dogmatic, but rather can become a helpful friend along the path of illness and recovery, enabling you to think in lateral ways about the whys and wherefores of being constantly below par, and how to cope better day-to-day with this state of affairs.

It is written by a fellow sufferer who has worked for the last 13 years to find solutions to becoming healthier, both in mind and body. Having had training in both nursing and midwifery and then at a later stage become a Masseuse and Reflexologist, I am conversant with modern medical techniques and practices. I share some of the things that have and haven't worked for me, emphasising that no two people are the same and what works for one may not be helpful for another. I have tried to gather information and tips from many sources; books, magazines, radio, TV and fellow sufferers.

Setting up a Fibromyalgia Support Group locally, I notice that often people are wary of sitting in a small group sharing intimate details of their health with relative strangers, and becoming a 'sufferer'. Some may prefer to read quietly in the privacy of their homes and ponder on things themselves.

Our paths are all unique and the reasons we are physically unwell are as unique as we are. These reasons I will explain more fully.

The online support sites set up by Fibromyalgia sufferers, where one reads about people's day-to-day struggles, make one realise how very many people are trapped in their illness, unable to go out at all, or have any sort of 'normal' life. In America there are now 12 million Fibromyalgics! In Britain the number quoted are about 1.2 million, and yet it is still one of the most ignored and mistreated illnesses by the NHS.

I am fortunate that I have always had the means of keeping the condition at a level where I can function, albeit often not as fully as I would wish. Over the last 13 years since I have been unwell I have learnt to look after myself, changing my life radically to support my weird body and learning what does and doesn't work. Sometimes I imagine I am 'better' until I push myself too hard and regress into tiredness and symptoms of pain and sleeplessness.

My greatest hope in writing this book is to give you a 'Toolbox' that you can dip into from time to time and that you will find a few new ideas to help you on your way. You may have friends and family who can benefit too. There is no need for people to suffer through ignorance. So many people in our society today are abusing their bodies unnecessarily.
Good luck with your process and I hope can I support you as much as I can from the printed page!

Disclaimer.

All the information in this book is for educational purposes only. It is not a substitute for medical advice, and the author and publishers accept no responsibility for any omissions or inaccuracies, errors or misstatements in the contents.

You are strongly encouraged to make your own health-care decisions based on your own research in partnership with qualified health-care professionals.

Any suggestions made here are inappropriate for young children and infants.

Angela Bea
2012.

Chapter 1. Illness and Dis-ease.

The term 'dis-ease' describes exactly what is happening to us when our bodies, emotions, minds and higher 'life purpose,' or that which we aspire to in our ideals, are out of harmony with one another. We are in some way unhappy, fearful, stuck or stressed on a deep psychological level and this becomes gradually reflected in our health. We are somehow out of balance in ourselves.

All illness is caused by dis-ease, although sometimes it is hard to spot the link between our lives and our health and it is not normal to look at this when we go to the GP or Consultant for a diagnosis and some pills or an operation to 'make it better.'

Fibromyalgia, Chronic Fatigue conditions and ME are becoming increasingly common in modern western medicine. These conditions may confuse and disempower our doctors unless they are very insightful and believe totally in the 'mind-body connection'.

Doctors themselves are trained in physical systems, symptoms and pathology. In medical training in the West we think of the body going wrong, rather like a car that breaks down and has to be mended. It is the Eastern systems of medicine, such as Ayuveda, and Chinese Medicine that teach us to look at things more holistically.

Autoimmune disorders and illnesses with allergies and unclear symptoms that cannot be categorized easily are now fairly common in our society. Why?

Modern living has become ever more STRESSFUL. We have lost touch with what is normal Healthy Living.

We drive around in cars, breathing in toxic fumes. Instead of exercising our bodies we sit in a traffic jam producing adrenaline from frustration and a 'fight, flight, fright' response which was developed by our ancestors to cope with being chased by a woolly mammoth or sabre toothed tiger!

We sit at computers for hours and strain our eyes, using fine muscles and nerve responses. Some get Repetitive Strain Injury but others just carry on unconcerned. There seems to be a huge increase in the numbers of people with Alzheimer's disease. Is this linked in any way?

We watch violent films and videos, again producing adrenaline from fear which is intended to activate our muscles but we do not go out for a brisk run, but rather we have a glass of wine and crash into bed.

We eat food which has been grown thousands of miles from where we live and has had large quantities of chemicals sprayed over it, before being irradiated 'to keep it fresh', flown in an aeroplane, wrapped in plastics, kept chilled, stored for weeks sometimes in our fridges/freezers Then it is micro waved, and reheated again. This is often called a 'normal healthy diet'. We have lost the connection between the earth/sun Energy that nourishes our cells in the food we eat. We 'poison' ourselves literally every day by eating food that is too dense and dead to contain any 'Life Energy'.

Obesity has now become the single greatest killer in the West. It seems as though we are unable to stop 'comfort eating' and overloading our bodies with heavy toxic matter which does not nourish, but is stored as fat and weighs us down. America and now Britain has an 'epidemic' of eating disorders.

Through our modern lifestyle we are stressing our human bodies to an extreme every day in every way and some people's bodies are less able to cope with this than others.

Why should some people get sick quicker than others? We all have a genetic inheritance. What our parents did and suffered also affects us profoundly. It is true that the 'sins of the father shall be meted upon the sons, through seven generations', as quoted from the Bible. Did our parents have stressful lives and suffer malnutrition? Certainly last century there were two World Wars to contend with. There were also more infectious illnesses. TB is one example, and drugs were used differently to treat illness. Large amounts of x rays were used also.

It is interesting to take a brief family history for yourself, going back 2-3 generations on both sides and see what effects you are dealing with in your genetic inheritance. It seems that some illnesses such as cancer and arthritis are not directly inherited but seem to cause a weakness in the immune system nevertheless.

What were you fed on as a child? Were you a post-war baby, encouraged to enjoy sweets, ice cream, school milk and orange juice? It is a concerning thought to think about the health of the nation in 40 years time considering the average diet of the modern child.

Meat and dairy now contain growth hormones and antibiotics, as a normal fact; vegetables are heavily sprayed with herbicides and fertilisers, even drinking water is polluted with these and also hormones from women on the pill. Small wonder then that our children are taller, denser and fatter, and going into puberty earlier.

Inoculations, vaccinations and immunizations cause our bodies to react as if we have a minor form of the illness. Instead of strengthening our immune systems it seems to have the effect of confusing and weakening our immunity if we have a lot of vaccinations at one time, especially as a young child or if we are stressed.

'Vacinosis' is a serious but largely unrecognised condition caused by mass vaccines, when the immune system goes into shut down. [It is recognised in veterinary practices and by naturopaths, but not by most doctors.] I had to have many vaccines before travelling abroad in 1997. A year later I started getting the symptoms of Fibromyalgia; an interesting link that may be connected?

Our minds and bodies are intrinsically linked together in all that we do. Our minds like to be in control of our lives. We like to be the boss of all we do. If our lives are ruled by others or we feel disempowered for any reason [bullied at work, or in an unhealthy relationship] we can become stressed. This is particularly seen in those who are 'passive aggressive', who hold the stress inside, resentful and angry that they are unable to take control of their own lives. Many Fibromyalgics live by the words 'ought' or 'should'!

Mental stress takes many forms and what is stressful for one may not be so for another. There are many factors involved in how we feel. Do our family and friends support us? How is our marriage, our finances, or our housing situation? Modern life tends to increase these stresses vastly.

Taking a look at your own life over the last few years, ask yourself where things have been difficult and where you have felt 'out of control'. It is quite well documented that ME can be triggered by stress, especially in workaholics! Are you a personality type A or B [i.e do you take a lead or remain as a supporter]? Do you take on others problems, are you the family supporter, are you trapped in an unhappy relationship? Are your fear patterns the result of your own parents' FEAR?

Self-knowledge is a great path to self-healing, as we gradually become aware of our patterns and weaknesses and FORGIVE these of ourselves and others. After all, none of us are perfect and we can perhaps ask why we are here on this earth at all? Are we here to learn lessons through our mistakes?

Illness gives us the perfect opportunity for reflection, as we have time to look at our lives, take stock and decide how to progress further. While we are sick we cannot rush around in action but have to stay peacefully 'looking at our navels' for a while, and this can bring real personal growth and enlightenment in it.

Whatever your personal view on the reason for your life here on earth, we can possibly all agree that illness is in itself a teacher, and from that perspective alone may be embraced with gratitude as we struggle day-to-day with all its implications and difficulties.

Health is the perfect, optimal situation for living out our lives, but if we suffer ill health then acceptance is the first step to healing ourselves, gratitude being the second.

We all have the power to change and hopefully with this toolkit you will feel inspired to have a go.

Chapter 2. What do we mean by Fibromyalgia, ME and Chronic Fatigue Syndrome?

This chapter is primarily for the use of those who stand around us; our family, friends, carers and the medical profession.

It is easy to go to the doctor with a list of symptoms about a chest infection, or a stomach upset or even depression, but when you feel constantly unwell and sometimes very ill, how do you compile a list of symptoms that will give a clear diagnosis to the doctor and not leave him and yourself at best feeling confused and at worst that he has a total hypochondriac sitting in front of him!

You could first try making a list of symptoms, starting from the top of the body working down, making it as detailed as possible, even if you don't get every symptom every day! Take this list with you to your appointment and refer to it in your conversation with the doctor.

As a Fibromyalgia sufferer I went to my GP initially thinking I had had winter 'flu, but wasn't getting any better. I just felt ill and achy all the time. My list of symptoms was changeable like the weather but nothing showed up on blood tests or urine samples. On one occasion my ESR [Erythrocyte Sedimentation Rate, which indicates an inflammatory process] was slightly raised but nothing else was conclusive until I went to the Rheumatology consultant 4 years later! I eventually insisted on this, suspecting I had Fibromyalgia, having read an American book about it that a friend had leant me. He pressed his fingers hard into several places on my back and I nearly shot through the roof! That was my definitive diagnosis [see diagram on front page.]

The diagnostic 'Tender Spots' are now the thing which they use most often to distinguish it from other conditions, and which gives one a **label**. How useful a label is, depends on how severely you are affected but it may enable you to get Disability Living Allowance or other benefits and can be the key to financial survival if you cannot work at all [although Fibromyalgia is noted a recognised and listed condition according to the DHSS!]

Financial aspects of being ill are in themselves very stressful and it is important to get support and advice to help you though this maze of beaurocracy.

Defining Fibromyalgia from other conditions is also important. Some similar conditions which ARE treatable and diagnosable are;

- Lyme's disease [a long-term bacteria from tick bites]
- Lupus Erythematosus [an autoimmune disease.]
- Polymyalgia [a form of rheumatism, mainly affecting neck and shoulders, treatable by steroids]
- Chronic systemic Candida [an overgrowth of fungus]
- Rheumatoid arthritis.
- Various more unusual osteoarthritic conditions, causing muscles to spasm.
- Hyper mobility, collagen disease [a lack of collagen in the connective tissue]
- Scleroderma [an autoimmune skin disease.]
- Abnormalities of the hormones and endocrine system.

This list is not definitive, but gives a broad sweep of some of the tests the doctors may perform, when you are being diagnosed.

The Fibromyalgia symptoms,

[Any, all, or a few of these can make for a confusing picture!]

- Muzzy head and dull thinking, 'brain fog', forgetting words mid-sentence, feeling spaced out and very tired. Depression can be mild or severe and be mixed with anxiety.
- Inability to have proper nights sleep, often staying most of the night in a dreamy sleep [level 3 sleep, whereas we all need level 4 deep sleep], waking early or for periods in the night. Restless legs. Waking up feeling tired and unrefreshed. Apnoea attacks are not uncommon [where the person stops breathing in their sleep.]
- Headaches are common.
- Tired dry scratchy eyes. Changeable vision.
- Trigeminal neuralgia [pain in the face, jaw], which can become very severe at times. Sensitive teeth.
- Stiff painful neck and shoulders, tender bruised feeling to the touch.
- **Any** muscles and joints can become painful and this tends to be worst first thing in the morning and can move around from limb to limb, found equally on both sides of the body, staying days or weeks in one spot. It can make

you feel like you have 'flu, and at worst you can hardly move at all. At best it feels sore and bruised to the touch.
- The **tender spots** which are located at the base of the skull, on the shoulders [midway between neck and shoulder joints] and over the inner rim of shoulder blades, just above the elbows, on the outer buttocks, on the hip bones, on the inner knees, just below the collar bone, and on the breast bone, all located evenly right and left, are the places where pain can be excruciating when pressed, indicative of muscle toxins building up and are diagnostic of Fibromyalgia. Interestingly they echo almost exactly some acupuncture spots, indicating a congested system on an Energetic level.
- Digestive problems are common; nausea, bloating and wind, IBS, sensitivities to many foods, which can even become severe allergies. Leaky gut syndrome, where inappropriate food molecules leak across into the blood stream from an inflamed or damaged small intestine. Sticky foul stools.
- Dry skin. Sensitivities to chemicals, creams, sun exposure and mosquito bites. Eruptions, psoriasis.
- Mild sore throats, furred tongue.
- Hypersensitivity to smells, especially diesel fumes, paints, smoke, etc.
- Hypersensitivity to lights, especially strip or blinking lights.
- Hypersensitivity to sounds or buzzing of electric equipment, fridges, heating systems, computers etc.

These are the most common symptoms and some or all may be present at any time. As one client beautifully describes it; 'The pain goes travelling on holiday and may end up anywhere!'

Many of the symptoms of ME are similar but without the tender spots. In this condition, as in Chronic Fatigue and also Gulf War Syndrome, there is an immense tiredness that can be so severe that muscles will not function at all and the person is confined to bed completely. In this situation the life energy of the person ceases to **be integrated** into the physical body so that the person only feels half alive. Lethargy and depression are often present and a general inability to function normally.

Exhaustion and stress can be a precursor to any of these more serious conditions and is a warning that the body is going into a sickness state. It should be an alert to take a time of complete rest and refreshment as the adrenals may have become affected and cannot respond normally to stress situations.

Long-term stress seems to be at the start of many of these conditions. The adrenal functions are finely tuned in us and also affect the other body hormones such as the female reproductive cycles, the thyroid, thymus, hypothalamus, pancreas and the pituitary [the master gland]. As we are all one integrated whole, an imbalance or stress on one part of the body will cause repercussions on other parts.

The nervous system also becomes debilitated in this state of stress/exhaustion, giving rise to the symptoms of tiredness, depression and foggy brain, as well as an oversensitivity and malfunction of perception of pain. Many people would define Fibromyalgia as a neurological condition.

When getting a definitive diagnosis it is important to exclude other illnesses [as listed above, and others]. Blood tests, urinalysis, MRI scans and other more complex testing can do this. The doctors may refer you to a specialist, a rheumatologist, endocrinologist or even a psychiatrist!

The actual causes of Fibromyalgia are still being debated. The body being so complex it has been suggested that hormones, the nervous system, viruses, post viral illnesses, toxins and stress may all be contributory. Often Fibromyalgia goes hand in hand with another condition such as Diabetes or Arthritis or chronic migraines, or may result from an acute accident or trauma.

Whatever the cause, the picture is that of the body collapsing and no longer functioning in the normal way, creating chronic pain, tiredness and malfunction of both the nervous system and the metabolic system.

Part of the frustration of having an illness like this can be a helplessness and lack of direction to get treatment. The doctors with their busy surgeries can only give support within a limited timescale and often make you feel you are a time waster. Reading around the subject can be invaluable at empowering you for further tests or discussions with the doctors.

When life is a struggle just to make a meal, and get up in the morning and your brain feels muzzy, reading a medical tome can be the last thing you can manage, so I have deliberately kept this book short and easy to refer to.

One can get completely bogged down with trying this that and the other, as a drowning man clutches at straws. It is better to try and keep it **simple** and look at the bigger picture. Why are you stressed and why has the body got ill? What can YOU do yourself to improve these things by how you eat, exercise, live, think and feel?

Have **trust** that YOUR BODY WILL HEAL ITSELF given the right time and environment, food and love. All these different systems, theories and treatments are only part of the bigger picture of who you truly are in essence and how you want to live out your life here on earth. Our illness can be the teacher of how to live in harmony with our beautiful planet, something that we have generally forgotten about in our modern day living. The earth itself is sick and needs our help too.

The path of healing can become a path of 'holism', by which I mean finding a balance of the body, mind and spirit and our relationship to the greater whole.

Chapter 3. Dehydration, cell health, acidity and alkalinity.

Our bodies, if normally healthy, are largely made up of water. Interestingly this is in the same proportion as the oceans to the land on this planet Earth! Water is vital for every function at a cellular level of our bodies. Without water we quickly die.

The interchange of all substances, food and minerals at a cellular level is dependent on the quality of this water. Electric currents which are vital in the fine interchange of substances at a microscopic level in our cells cannot flow properly in 'stagnant' water. Therefore it is important to look at how the body is maintaining and cleansing itself at this level.

Acids are formed by the breakdown of certain foods [and also by what we call stress.] Therefore foods are categorised as being acid or alkaline. Eating alkaline foods is a good way to start healing. **People with Fibromyalgia are over-acid.**

Dr Robert Young, an American Biochemist, whom I have met, in his book 'The pH Miracle' describes this process and gives a list of alkaline foods. There is also a very comprehensive English web site now available on alkalizing [energiseforlife.com], which lists foods and their potential pH quality [see Appendix 1.]

Barbara Wren has written a very excellent book called 'Cellular Awakening'. In it she describes the stagnation of disease and how we can come to a place of health. I cannot recommend this book too highly. She runs the College of Natural Nutrition [www.natnut.co.uk], which would be a good place to search for help on dietary changes and supplements.

It is very interesting to note that in a healthy cell there is a day/night rhythm of interchange of the substances sodium/calcium and lipids [good fats] and magnesium/potassium. In Fibromyalgia this process is disturbed, hence waking up feeling tired! Our cells have not been properly cleansed overnight because of DEHYDRATION, creating a build up of toxins in the body and hence the pain in the tissues/muscles and the foggy brain feeling. We are literally TOXIC.

The first place to start therefore is by detoxifying.

Nowadays there is much written in magazines about healthy eating and detoxing. It is nearly all good healthy advice. What needs to be said however is that the body is in shutdown in Fibromyalgia and any extreme cleanse will only put more stress on it. Doing anything too radically and quickly creates too much poison circulating in the body fluids and the kidneys and lymphatic systems cannot cope. Decide therefore how and what you are going to do and get it checked out and supported if possible by a nutritional therapist.

Common sense and enthusiasm need to be backed up with knowledge when you have a sick body!

Another way to start becoming more alkaline and to detoxify is to invest in a **water ioniser** that connects to the tap in the kitchen. Drink **at least** 2 pints of this special alkaline water a day. This is a basic water filter and takes out all impurities and chemicals, as well as giving the actual water a lower pH level, so it goes more easily into each cell and rehydrates them. It is an expensive investment but can be hired on a monthly basis first to try it out.

If you can start to think of your body as needing special care and attention - **good food, fresh air, relaxation, and exercise** - you can start to plan how you are going to get from a place of illness with a diagnosis of an incurable chronic condition which is little understood [almost a death sentence!] to a place of health, wellbeing and contentment, even if this means completely rethinking your life as it is now and changing the way you eat, live and even you emotions and thoughts, which also can cause toxicity and acidity in the body.

That is the theory, now onto the practical details of HOW to do it!

Chapter 4. Good food.

Food needs to be enjoyed first and foremost, as it is our way of connecting ourselves to planet earth. Our bodily substance is made up of what we eat. Cooking a meal, shopping and planning menus can become a real chore and a struggle when you are feeling rough and achy, as you probably do most of the time, so it is important to keep it simple. But it is the most important thing that we can change ourselves, on our path to healing and if we get this right we can start to feel in charge of our own lives again.

As Fibromyalgia is a condition very closely associated with toxicity, it is of the utmost importance to try and **cleanse** your body as much as you can. One can also try and rid the body of some of its excess acidity.

These dietary suggestions are for your new life, not just to try for a few weeks. A complete change of eating habits may take a little while to get used to, so introduce new foods gradually and experiment with different things that may be new to you. Try not to get obsessive or anxious about it all, as that can create acid thoughts too, which in turn creates more toxins. Don't become afraid of food! If you do a radical detox you may get headaches for a couple of days as the cells cleanse and all the toxins circulate around your body. Drink extra water to 'flush them out' and allow your body to rest an extra amount, as it otherwise will add stress. Ideally do not do anything radical!

There are many excellent websites and books on dietary changes. You may become interested in this vast subject, but initially do not get overwhelmed by everyone's research and knowledge. Keep it simple.

Foods to avoid.

In order to detoxify the body try to **avoid** these substances from day 1.

Always read the labels! Learn to say 'No thanks' when out and about!

Monosodium Glutamate [found in many highly flavoured foods, instant soups, sauces, crisps, Chinese meals.] This has been found to be highly poisonous to some individuals, and may cause muscle spasms as well as headaches or tummy upsets.

Aspartame, found in artificial sweeteners, many low calorie drinks, and sugar free chewing gum. This substance can also accumulate in the body tissues and in America where low sugar fizzy drinks [e.g. diet coke] are consumed in large quantities young people have been showing symptoms similar to Multiple Sclerosis.

Caffeine, found in tea, coffee, coke, chocolate and some high energy drinks. This over stimulates the nervous system, causing sleep disturbances, muscle spasms and palpitations or hot flushes and is a complete poison to anyone with Fibromyalgia. Decaffeinated coffee and tea are <u>not</u> good substitutes as most of the decaffeinating process involves the use of toxic chemicals as well.

Sugar, especially sucrose. The use of sweets and added sugar as well as cakes and preserves is undoubtedly connected with an increase in type two diabetes in our society and also fungal growth in our bodies. Often in Fibromyalgia, when the whole body has been stressed and the adrenals, insulin production and thyroid are out of balance, excess sugar can lead to the condition of Candida throughout the body, which causes leaky gut and toxins in the muscles, lungs and brain, giving symptoms of Fibromyalgia. It is better therefore to assume that there is Candida around when detoxing and cut out most sugars. A little honey, dates, or natural sugars from fruit can be used sometimes, especially if you have sweet cravings, which will gradually change as you start to rebalance your tastes. You could try agave and rice syrup too, or liquid fructose. It is better though to rely on the natural sweetness in vegetables to satisfy our need for this taste.

Alcohol and low-alcohol substitutes. This may seem radical for some but alcohol is extremely toxic to a sick body, especially the additives put into wine making. Once you are cleansed you may want to perhaps try an occasional glass of organic wine and see how your muscles respond.

Colourings and flavourings and other additives. These are added to very many foodstuffs nowadays and become cumulative in the body. ALWAYS READ THE LABELS and try if possible to cook meals only made from fresh organic ingredients that will contain nothing but the odd slug or greenfly!

<u>Mind altering drugs of any kind, including prescribed medicines.</u> It may take some time before you are ready to come off prescribed painkillers or antidepressants if you are taking them, but make this your final aim, as long-term use of these create toxins also and can suppress your brain activity. Recent research indicates that they may also contribute to the development of Alzheimer's disease. Many people go to their GPs for help and are prescribed large amounts of allopathic drugs. We have become a society of pill poppers. It can be frightening to walk your path alone with a chronic illness, which is why it is so important to get the support of friends, family and good therapists who can walk along beside you on your path of Healing. Keep communications open with your doctor though as you never now when you will need their help and guidance. Reducing your medication is the first step, but do this with medical guidance, especially steroids and antidepressants.

<u>Giving up smoking</u> is a vital part of your healing, but may need professional support, hypnotherapy etc. Take it a step at a time once you are feeling a bit better. Nicotine, like other artificial substances, acts as a strong toxin in the body. It also effects the peripheral circulation and has a similar effect to an adrenaline rush, which your body may crave if it is exhausted, but does NOTHING to help you to heal.

<u>General help for the metabolic system.</u>

Gradually introduce more and more fibre into your diet and use the foods listed as **Alkaline** in the Appendix. The acid/alkaline balance must be considerably changed to reduce the symptoms of Fibromyalgia.

If you do this too quickly you may find you are windy or get loose stools. Don't fear, just ease off a little and persevere. Your body WILL adapt and gradually the minute Villae in your small intestines, damaged by poor food quality and stress, will heal. This can take months, depending on the severity of your condition.

Try to buy **Organic fruit and vegetables** whenever possible. This may be a little more expensive but it is money well worth spending, as chemical sprays that accumulate in soil [and also deplete the soil of other trace elements that are vital to healthy bodily functions] are extremely poisonous to sensitive bodies. If you cannot buy organic food at local shops, try getting food from a local farmer's market or order a weekly box online from a company such as Riverford's, who will deliver lovely fresh local grown produce.

A good rule of thumb is to try and eat at least 2/3rd of a plate of vegetables at each main meal [lunch and supper]. This can be as salads, or lightly steamed, stir-fried or oven roasted vegetables [using slow cooking so as not to burn the olive oil.]

Eating a variety of different colours of food means that you have variety of minerals and vitamins, so pick a rainbow selection and eat a little of many kinds of vegetables grown locally and as seasonal as possible. Try to leave them in the fridge for a minimal time, as each day they sit there they 'die' and lose some energy. By doing this you are taking in the greatest number of Vitamins and Trace Mineral elements as possible, and also linking your body's energy to local Earth energy which is healing in itself.

Of course the very best food is that dug straight out of your garden. Maybe you can look forward to a time when this will become possible, even if now it doesn't seem likely. Raised beds and no dig methods means that once set up they take very little physical energy to cultivate. Herbs, which are particularly rich in minerals and vitamins, are a good place to start. Keep a few handy on the kitchen windowsill.

An interesting and 'Holistic' way of planning a meal is to think of eating all the different parts of the plant in one meal. This could include a root vegetable [e.g. carrot], a stem [e.g. celery], a leaf [some green salad or fresh herbs], a flower [e.g. broccoli, borage, marigold], some seeds or nuts [pumpkin, sunflower, almonds, walnuts, pine nuts], and some fruit. The qualities of all these parts are different and in Macrobiotic terms contain a good balance of Yin and Yang Energy [expansion and contraction of energetic substance.] Some contain high protein, and stored energy; some have more sugars and give you instant energy.

We have been led to believe that a 'good diet' contains carbohydrates, proteins and fats [and that we should not eat too many of the latter!], minerals and vitamins. I will look at each of these elements separately.

Interestingly all these substances can be found in a purely vegan diet, in the different parts of the plant!

Carbohydrates

These are starchy foods, and give us long lasting energy. They are broken down less quickly than true sugars, and therefore act as 'coke on a slow burning furnace.' It is important that we eat a certain amount of these, but many people nowadays are becoming intolerant of gluten, found in wheat most especially. It can cause irritable bowel syndrome, wind and inflammation in the small intestine. Often if we leave wheat out for a while and concentrate on healing the gut with organic cooked vegetables and rice or Quinoa then we can reintroduce organic cereals gradually after a while with no ill affect. It is primarily the chemical sprays on the cereals that we become allergic to.

In Britain the staple food is **bread,** often using highly refined white flour with many additives, flour improvers and very little food value. The sprays used in wheat production go into the grain head more easily than most other grains, so could it be the fertilizers, which are causing the sudden increase of 'gluten intolerance'?

Try replacing wheat bread with rice cakes, oat cakes, sour dough rye bread, yeast free 'Village Bakery' rye bread, pumpernickel from Germany [some varieties have wheat in them], delicious but expensive 'sprouted grain bread' available in whole food shops, or try making your own soda bread with a variety of non-wheat organic flours and wheat free soda. Spelt bread is made from an ancient form of wheat and may be better tolerated. The slow-rising, double knead method of bread making is more easily digested. Alternatively replace the 'sandwich meal' with a mixed vegetable salad and add some cooked brown rice or buckwheat/ rice pasta, seasoned with herbs - delicious!

Try to start each day with a Carbohydrate meal. This gives you plenty of fuel after the fast of the night and will sustain you until lunch, except for fluid. This could be muesli, made from organic mixed grains, avoiding wheat, and added organic seeds, sweetened with some fresh fruit pieces such as berries. It is best to soak the grain for 15 minutes or so to release toxins found in raw oats. This also makes it easier to digest. Or you could make some porridge if it is a cold day, which warms the digestive tract.

First Class Proteins.

It is a matter of preference whether one is a meat eater, fish eater, eggs and dairy eater, but these all contain first class proteins, and as such are known as 'essential' to a healthy diet. If you choose to reduce the amounts of these proteins in the diet, you can be equally healthy as a vegan, either strict or partial. However it is very important then to consume enough **vegetable protein**, as protein is converted into amino acids, the building blocks for new cell growth. Vegetarian proteins [2nd class proteins] should include combinations of pulses with seeds or nuts, grains with pulses, or grains with nuts/seeds. These are known as second-class proteins. There are many vegetarian recipe books on this subject available.

If you do decide to stay as a meat eater, try to **reduce the amount** you eat by at least half, as meat [and all first class proteins] is very acidic and therefore do not help achy muscles and joints. It is important also to source organic meat, which can be very expensive.

Fish is also not without its problems. Heavy metals, such as mercury, are found in high doses in some deep-sea fish, and these can be toxic to a sensitive body. Small oily fish such as sardines, mackerel and sprats are best to eat regularly. Try to eat these at least twice a week.

The debate of WHAT one eats is complex and comes down to life-style, constitution and family habits. To change radically overnight could throw the body into shock, so make any long-term changes gradually. Just keep in mind the acid levels and the toxins in inorganic meat, fish, milk and egg production.

Becoming a vegetarian certainly makes one feel 'lighter' and more energised. For some though it can be an ungrounding experience, so you feel floaty and unreal. Try it for yourself.

Dairy Foods
Many people with Fibromyalgia become allergic to dairy products. Again, this is largely due to the foodstuffs that the cows are fed on including hormones and antibiotics. Try replacing milk with organic Soya, rice or almond milk. Yoghourt, which helps stabilize the gut flora, is important too. It is available as goat's or Soya yoghourt. Organic goat's cheeses, feta and cottage cheeses are available too. Some allergic people can tolerate organic goats milk and yoghourt, and even organic cottage cheese, others don't. All these products are now widely available in supermarkets. You may find you can occasionally tolerate a little organic cow's milk or yoghourt at a later stage. 'Quark' and fromage

frais is tolerated by most people and a good source of protein, but too much will make you acidic.

Fats
These are vital for our health. Much is written these days about 'bad fats' and cholesterol rising, causing heart disease and strokes. Cholesterol is not a DIRECT result of eating fat, but a much more complex process, often as a result of too much stress.

If you cut out fats altogether, as some Slimming clubs would have us do, the cell walls have no building blocks and one can become very ill. Instead ensure you have enough GOOD FATS.

These include olive oils, hemp, sunflower, walnut, sesame, etc., in fact a large variety of organic vegetable oils. It is interesting to note that the Omegas, which we read so much about now, differ according to where the plant grows. In our colder climate we need mainly Omega 3; as we move south towards the Mediterranean the oils have more Omega 6; in hot climates they have Omega 9.

One can therefore adjust the type of Omega according to season and temperature, adding oily fish in the winter, and eating lighter oils in the summer.

Vitamins and Minerals.
These substances are vital in small amounts for healthy cell function. For example Magnesium gives the cells the 'light' quality to refresh and cleanse. Nowadays factory farming does much harm to the soils and erosion from wind and rain,

coupled with the use of inorganic fertilizers, means that the plants themselves do not contain the vital nutrients that our bodies need for health.

Therefore you may need to take some supplements, at least initially. Some books on Fibromyalgia have confusingly long lists of high dose supplements, which are maybe not necessary.

Using Supplements has become common practice and until recent EU directives on the certification of all medicines, [which has meant some companies have gone out of business because of the high cost of legalising a product,] these were readily available over the counter in both pharmacies and supermarkets. The staff in Whole food shops are generally more knowledgeable and can often advise on their use and dosage, but it is probably best to search out a recommended nutritionalist to get this highly complicated subject sorted out.

The body normally excretes any excess supplements, but in a state of toxicity, which already exists, high doses may make the matter worse.

Generally Vitamin C, B complex [especially B6 and B12] and **magnesium** are supplements that the body requires in Fibromyalgia, but there may be other vital ones missing, such as Zinc, so try to get help on this vast science.

Many excellent books have been published [see Appendix 3] where you can go in depth and learn about different supplements and their actions. This book is for simple self-help techniques only.

There are several different ways you can be tested to see if you need Vitamin and Mineral supplements. Check this on a website of 'mineral and vitamin testing' to read about live and dried blood analysis, and tasting mineral kits.

Chapter 5. What can I eat and drink?

With such a long list of 'No no's' you may well be wondering what is left to eat!

Fruit and vegetables, as mentioned before, make up the bulk of your new diet, but many other things can be added for a good mixed diet.

Beverages.

Herbal teas are now widely available and are becoming more normal in cafes and homes. Always carry a few spare ones with you in case you get caught out.

The fruit mixtures are generally not good because they contain artificial flavourings. Tea from fresh leaves is best, made in a china pot, and allowed to infuse for 5-7 minutes before sipping slowly.

A recently published list of the best alkalising teas included:
-

Roibosch [red bush tea from South Africa], which can become a good substitute to your English cup of tea, made fairly strong, with Soya or rice milk added. If you are used to sweet tea, try the Soya milk with apple juice until you are more used to it. It can also be drunk black.

Matte tea makes a pleasant drink and is good for you either with or without milk.

Peppermint tea is good after a meal to help digestion. There are various mixtures available, or use fresh leaves.

Detox mixtures are helpful, including ones using fennel and other herbs.

Ginger and lemon cleanses and stimulates the digestion.

A calming 'sleepy time' mixture can be good to sip at bedtime.

Try growing a few yourselves, including sage, good for bad throats and winter colds; thyme, another warming tea; marjoram, cleansing; chamomile, for tummy upsets and lemon balm, refreshing if allowed to cool for a hot day. Rosemary is warming to the system and enlivens the circulation; lemon verbena is also very refreshing, but susceptible to winter frosts.

An herb garden outside the back door can be a wonderful place to quietly go and watch the bees buzzing and smell the different aromas. Planting lavender nearby is also helpful for a stressed body and mind.

Coffee substitutes.

Many people miss their morning cup of coffee. The thicker substance of this milky drink can be sustaining and comforting, whereas herb teas are thinner and more thirst quenching.

In the health food shops you find a variety of coffee substitutes, including Yanno, Barley Cup, No Caf and Dandelion coffee mixtures. Instant powders are easiest to use, but dandelion root ground up and brewed for 7-10 minutes makes a dark bitter coffee mixture that is strained and milk added, and is an excellent liver cleanser.

Coffee gives the mind a clarity which you may crave in Fibromyalgia and gives the 'kick-start' energy for the day, but don't be tempted to take a short-term fix which will further weaken your system, and delay your healing.

Water and juices.

If you are unable to afford an Ioniser, which gives you alkaline water, try to drink spring water but only out of glass bottles. Plastics used for bottled water give off toxins, especially if kept in a warm place in the sun. Drink as much as you can, as the pure water flushes out toxins and often dehydration is a basic cause for ill health.

Each person's body is different in its need for daily water. It depends on the climate, central heating, activity, renal function, amount of fat in the body, the state of the cells and fluids themselves and amount of salt consumed.

The salt/water ratio is controlled in the kidneys and as long term dehydration and too much salt have often stressed these, it is important to LISTEN to your own body. Are you thirsty? When? Is your urine pale and clear [healthy] or dark and strong smelling? If you pick up the skin on the back of your hand is it lose or firm? Does it rebound?

Some books recommend x amount of water to be drunk daily. Do not take this too literally if you have any kind of congestion in your circulation as you may make it worse. Reduce your salt intake gradually, using first rock salt, then 'low salt' if you need a little in cooking. As you get healthier your natural salt /water balance will improve and you will have a better sense of how much water you need to drink. Ideally you should aim at needing no salt addition at all.

Water should not be drunk with meals as it dilutes the digestive juices and saliva acts as an important first place where digestion starts as it mixes with the food. Instead have a glass near you and sip it throughout the day. Ideally don't drink anything half an hour before and 2 ½ hours after eating a main meal.

Drink extra water in hot weather, if you are going on a journey, especially flying, or if life gets a bit more stressful.
Fruit juices can be healthy if pure and organic. Avoid the cheap cartons of 'juice drink' as they contain large amounts of sugar and juice made from concentrate has little value as well. Only drink fruit juice instead of eating a fruit, best taken between meals, as the acid is less well digested as part of the main meal. Don't replace your water with fruit juices. One is vital to life; the other is a liquid food.

Many people are allergic to the sprays used in orchards and especially on oranges and grapefruits, and grapes. These fruits are best avoided at first unless organic.

Lemons are very ALKALISING for most people surprisingly as they seem very acid. A very healthy way to start the day is to drink the juice of half an organic lemon, mixed with some warm water, at least half an hour before breakfast. You can also use them liberally in salad dressings and just drizzled over vegetables. They lose Vitamin C quickly so fresh squeeze them and do not heat them unnecessarily. Cut a slice into your drinking water too. You may be someone who cannot metabolise these fruit acids into alkaline; trial and error is the best way to find out, with urine testing for pH.

Second class proteins.

As mentioned before proteins create essential building blocks for the cells, but unless you are consciously combining them together they do not create full amino acids and cannot be utilised fully by the body.

Nuts and seeds.

These can easily be freshly ground up in small quantities just prior to use in a small coffee grinder if you have any dental problems. They must otherwise be very well chewed, or else they can irritate an already sensitive small intestine.

Freshness is important. Check the sell-by date and only buy organic ones. Store nuts in screw top jars in a cool place, as they easily grow toxic moulds, which can be poisonous, so use them quickly.

Nuts and seeds can be eaten with grains to create 1st class protein, as on muesli, or added to vegetable meals and salads, where there are also pulses or grains. Good varieties are pumpkin, sunflower, linseed [which is especially good for healing the small intestines, soaked for a few hours] pine nuts, almonds [the most alkaline], walnuts and cashews and also chestnut purée and coconut milk or cream.

Pulses.

Some people can find these hard to digest so soak them thoroughly for several hours, and then rinse them well can get rid of the unwanted toxins, which create windiness.

Eat them occasionally in stews and soups, especially in winter, or cook some ready to create a mixed salad and keep in the fridge. Add a few lentils if cooking rice to go with curry, or have a simple meal of baked beans [organic low sugar variety] on wholemeal toast if you don't feel like cooking. Always be aware of combining them with a grain or nuts/seeds.

Soya is a good form of protein, and can be taken as milk, yoghourt, tofu curd or beans. Ensure you eat organic non GM varieties only. They are also helpful for balancing oestrogen in the menopause, but some people are allergic to them.

Grains

There are many grains that have been cultivated over centuries from wild grasses, and each has a different quality. As with the Omega oils, some are more suitable for hot climates, some for cold. They must all be well cooked and masticated to help digestion, as the carbohydrates need to be well mixed with saliva to start the breakdown of substances in the gut.

Try some of these: -

Barley, especially good as a winter stew, or as flour mixed with other grains in bread. It is warming to the digestion and especially good in winter.

Oats; porridge, muesli, flapjacks, crumble toppings, both sweet and savoury, contains toxins if eaten raw without some soaking. It is also warming to the system.

Wheat; bread, pancakes, cakes etc. Whole-wheat grains can be soaked and well cooked, seasoned with herbs and tamari as an accompaniment with vegetables. Wheat is our staple in the west, but causes problems for some as it holds artificial fertilisers in the kernels and has high gluten levels. Always use organic wholemeal flour to get the goodness. Cous cous and cracked wheat are varieties of wheat and useful alternatives to rice eaten with a main meal, providing you are not wheat intolerant. Spelt flour is made from an ancient type of wheat which is becoming more widely used again. It holds less chemicals in the denser head, and is often tolerated well when wheat causes allergies.

Buckwheat; as above, a nutty taste, and the flour makes super pancakes. Also very good for the circulation as it contains rutin, which strengthens vein walls.

Maize/corn; can be eaten straight off the cob as a vegetable, or as a flour, for thickening etc. Corn bread as made in America makes a nice variety if you are wheat free. Try making popcorn in a large saucepan for some fun.

Millet; this grows in long tendrils and is best known as budgerigar food, but is an extremely healthy grain from southern Europe and Africa. It contains silica and is a natural diuretic and cleanser. It needs fairly long, slow cooking and can be added to soups or served as a base for mixed vegetables. It is bland in taste so needs seasoning with fresh herbs. It can also be made into a milk pudding if cooked slowly in the oven.

Quinoa [pronounced keen-wa] or amaranth; this is a north American Indian grain which is becoming better known as is extremely healthy. It can be slow cooked as porridge, as an accompaniment for vegetables or as flour makes good nutty tasting cakes and scones, best blended with rice and Soya flour.

Rice; well known in Indian cooking, but brown rice is much more nutritious if well cooked. The husks which are removed in white rice contain B Vitamins. Rice flour is useful for baking and blends well with other flours. Brown rice is an excellent staple food if you are fasting and cleansing for a few days. Black wild rice is also a nice alternative.

With all grains long slow cooking is important and they can therefore become a bit of a chore to cook if you are not well. A 'hay-box', a highly insulated container into which you put the saucepan once it has come to the boil, or slow cooker, may be a way around this. However try out different grains and keep some in the fridge for instant high-energy food if you are very tired. Rice puddings, made without sugar, are easy to prepare and very comforting if you haven't much appetite. You can try a spoonful of sugar free jam on them for an extra treat!

Sprouted pulses, grains and seeds are very healthy and full of vitamins and minerals. Try growing some on your windowsill, in a special sprouter, and rinsing twice a day. Once they show green tips and long white roots they can be lightly stir-fried or added to salads, but be careful to rinse them off very thoroughly beforehand in running water, as they can contain toxins if not. You can also buy them fresh from the supermarket or whole-food shop, and again they will need thorough rinsing before use.

Treats.

We all like to treat ourselves to something tasty from time to time as a comfort if we are stressed or depressed and it is very easy to resort back to old habits of a bar of chocolate, a cream cake, a glass of wine, a packet of biscuits or a steak. Try to have a little store of healthy snacks to nibble on if you feel like this, so a small 'sin' is better than setting yourself back health wise and chastising yourself afterwards as you suffer all your old symptoms.

Some foods like this might include a mint carob sugar free bar [like chocolate, available in good health food shops]; sugar free fruit chewy bars, 85% or 70% organic chocolate [just a small piece!], 'Nakt' date bars, a really nice ripe mango or peach, some homemade fruit sorbet, a banana smoothy, some low salt organic crisps, some well washed organic dried fruit, a handful of cashew nuts. None of these are 'good' for you [except the fruit and nuts] but may stop you climbing the wall and feeling miserable and in small quantities should be all right.

This last chapter has gone into a lot of detail about food, the reason being that food and drink is the biggest single thing we have **control over** on our path to recovery. If you can concentrate on this chapter first you have a high chance of making some real changes in your health over time. Have patience and persevere. We are literally what we eat.

Chapter 6. Therapies and self-help treatments.

At a time when the medical world is becoming ever more technical and impressive it is a fact that more and more people are searching out and using Complementary Therapies; at least 20% of the population use them at any one time!

The word 'Complementary' as opposed to 'Alternative' indicates that the help we are seeking is perhaps a positive extra to our normal medical treatment. But how do they work?

If we look for a moment at the essence of life, the Atom, we see small particles of substance constantly moving around. This is the smallest known living thing and is directed by our DNA or inherited blueprint. What the scientists don't ask [but nowadays are investigating ever more] is what creates the movement or LIFE ENERGY in every living thing? Why do the particles move constantly? It is this movement which is being addressed in Therapies such as Homeopathy, Reflexology, Massage, Shiatsu, Yoga, Tai Chi, Healing, Reiki, Biofeedback, Zero Balancing, Cranio-sacral therapy, and many others.

All over the world there are ancient healing methods which recognise the body's own healing instinct. If a body is out of its own balance [and every body is unique and innately imbalanced!] then giving an 'intention of change' through precise movement from outside will help the body to rebalance itself. This may seem a difficult concept, but watch the potter change clay into a thing of beauty on the wheel and you can get an inkling of the process.

Added to this physical/energetic process of changing matter by ones very intention, you have also the unique interchange of two human beings in the 'Therapeutic process'; one who wishes to help and heal and the other who wants to be healed. Therapists have been deeply trained in 'enabling' others to change and grow.

The psychological aspect of Therapies has been well researched and has been found to have real value. Your treatment is a time set aside just for YOU, when you can talk and be heard, where you can learn to relax and evaluate your life journey and what part your illness plays in it all.

Many people with Fibromyalgia resort to having regular Complementary treatments of one kind or another. Here are just a few hints if you don't know what to look for.

- Look for someone through personal recommendation or on a professional website. Try and use only people who are on an official register of qualified practitioners.

- Make sure the treatment room allows you to be quiet and relaxed. Can you get there easily? Are there difficult stairs? Can they come and treat you at home? Do you like the atmosphere, the smell, the way the therapist welcomes you. Do you prefer a man or a woman therapist? Does it feel friendly, professional, unrushed, clean, and is it affordable? Can you cancel if you are not well? All these elements are important.

- Do you like being touched? All over? Just on your feet? Do you mind getting partially undressed? Get the therapist to explain the treatment and how it works before you go for your first session so you know what to expect.

- Do you want a one-to-one session, or would you rather do something yourself, like a Yoga, Tai-Chi or Pilates class, in a group?

As time goes on, you will start to feel a benefit. If for some reason it isn't helping you in ANY way, [and change can be subtle and slow sometimes,] then have a reappraisal with your Therapist to see where it is going. Are you feeling there is enough support and counselling? Are you physically warm and comfortable during treatments? How do you feel immediately afterwards? Sometimes there is a 'healing reaction' where you feel worse for a couple of days.

Chopping and changing around and trying lots of different therapies is not always helpful. Each therapy works in a slightly different way and the body can get confused by too much input. So stick with one for a while and then change if you are unhappy with it. It is frustrating for therapists too to feel you are shopping around or clutching at straws to get a quick fix recovery. There is no such thing when your body is Fibromyalgic!!

A therapeutic break is sometimes necessary for the body to respond to what it has been 'told'. Your therapist will advise you.

Self-help treatments at home.

1. Aromatherapy Baths. Get yourself a good book on aromatherapy and buy a few well chosen oils. Know when and how to use them as they can be very strong acting. Take time to enjoy a relaxing bath, either at night to help you to sleep or first thing in the morning to get your muscles going, when you are stiff and achy. Salts from the Dead Sea contain high Magnesium and are super to soak away the pains too.

2. Try dry brushing your skin before your daily bath/shower. This stimulates the circulation and lymph flow and helps excrete toxins from the skin. Start with your arms and legs and always brush towards the heart in brisk strong strokes.

3. Foot Massage. Buy some lovely natural cream preferably with lanolin or beeswax in it and give yourself a good deep foot massage. It is nearly as good as a Reflexology if you do it with loving care! You could try a nice warm footbath first to soften and warm everything up.

   4. Use ONLY natural substances on your skin. Go through all your cupboards and drawers and throw out the chemicals [make-up, perfumes, deodorants, hairsprays etc] which are making you sick and also not helping the planet. Some very good brands of skin care are available now using only plant oils and natural aromas [Weleda, Hauschka, and Faith in Nature for example].

5. Go through the cleaning cupboards and throw out or give away anything that has toxic chemicals in it and replace them with mild environmentally friendly ones. Ecover

products are good for cleaning. Remember that you are toxic, so everything in this direction is helping you to heal; you are not just becoming a health freak!

6. Try to clean up your wardrobe too. Organic cotton is best for underwear; avoid the use of synthetics where possible. They are not healthy for your skin and excretory system. Pure silk, soft wool and cotton are always best.

7. Use houseplants to help clean your house. Spider plants help absorb electro magnetic energy from computers! A variety of beautiful well cared for plants will increase the beauty and natural environment. Enjoy daily care of these too.

8. A clean house will not only cheer you up but has a very positive therapeutic effect. Old stale energy gets trapped in dust and grime and can even make you sick. If you are not on top of your cleaning, consider a blitz from friends or professionals to give you a boost start. Declutter your space, especially your bedroom and throw out anything you have not used for at least a year. This cleansing process WILL make a huge difference to your health and feeling of wellbeing.

9. Use crystals as 'friends' around the house. You may become interested in their powerful therapeutic effect too, but be careful to keep them clean as they will absorb lots of negative energy. Wash them in warm soapy water and rinse well then stand in sunshine or moonlight.

10. You may like to burn incense or have candles around. Some people find the smell overpowering, so perhaps limit their use to one or two rooms.

11. If you live as a couple or with children and find it difficult to get away from all the mess and noise try to find a corner which is just for you! It may mean negotiating a spare bedroom, attic space or even a garden room, but it is vital that you have somewhere quiet, clean and peaceful to rest and just BE. Ensure that this space is uncluttered, and does not have any electrical gadgets switched on, even at the plug. Keep some fresh flowers there if possible and a few books you can pick up if you want to read. Go there to rest in the day and enjoy your solitude. It is different from loneliness which can come from social isolation and living alone. In this situation consider getting a small pet for company. If you feel too unwell to join active groups, try to get out occasionally to a local Fibro self-help group or join a church, social club [not the heavy drinkers!] or singles club. Isolation can be very stressful. Look at your life and ask why you are alone. It is usually a defence mechanism which has separated you from others. Do you moan about life, or only talk about Me! Try to _give_ love and enjoy other people's busy lives. We are all different.

12. Finding creativity in your life is very healing and can reduce stress enormously. You may never have had the oportunity for this in your life before, so explore what you enjoy doing. Join a pottery group, an art class, embroidery group, woodwork, jewellery or card making group or even a creative writing group. Explain when you enrol that you have health problems so that the tutor is aware of your needs.

Each day is different. When you wake up, go and look outside and breathe deeply. Is it calm and sunny, windy or frosty, warm or cold? Listen to the sounds around you. Feel the air on your skin. Feel your feet on the ground and be grateful for a new exciting day ahead full of promise and creativity. What will today bring?

Use this space to list what makes YOU feel good!

Chapter 7. How to make life easier.

Living with Fibromyalgia can create a great sense of depression and anxiety; one can learn and practise simple techniques of harmonising your mind and body, and coming to a peaceful place of Acceptance. If you are less stressed about your condition mentally you will cope better and get less depressed generally.

Because your body has become weak and painful it stops you in your life tracks and allows you time to reconsider what you have been doing with your life up to this point and how to change this state of being. You are in a very privileged position that illness gives you, which you do not have if you are out in the fast track of life. You have been given TIME.

You can endlessly ask yourself WHY you are ill, and see your condition as literally a 'pain', where something is 'wrong' with you and it isn't going to get any better, but rather get worse as you get older. Many books on Fibromyalgia are written from this perspective, and it is also the attitude you may well find in the medical establishment, with the consultant Rheumatologist and the GP. Pain is usually a signal of the body that something is very wrong and needs mending. In Fibromyalgia the body gives out pain signals when it is still pretty fine except for a load of toxins, which MIGHT make you very ill eventually. It is warning you to change your habits and life direction. It is like a barometer as to how healthily and harmoniously you are living your life. If you do something wrong it will tell you! Now is our chance to change things!

Practicing Right Thinking can be about being conscious in the moment. It is about not worrying about tomorrow or regretting what has happened. It is about being fully PRESENT in today, now. The 'present' is literally a gift and we can become and practise being grateful for our current 'state of beingness.' Eckhart Tolle has produced a good meditation tape called 'Entering the NOW' which is helpful to work with.

Every day is different and every day you are becoming healthier. If you wake up one day and everything seems black and painful, look at yourself long and hard in the mirror, smile and say to your reflection "You are getting better every day, in every way. Everything is just PERFECT. You are doing really well. I love you." You may not believe that at first. But keep saying it and things gradually start to change for the better.

Something in you may not want to believe it. Maybe even be a tiny place in your subconscious says it serves you well to be ill, so that you can get more attention, care, love or money? That is an interesting thought! Look at it and be honest with yourself.

Emotional reaction to illness is part of the illness itself. This, like the food you eat, is another power tool for your toolkit. You have the POWER to change your thought patterns. It takes practice and patience but it DOES work. Is your glass half empty or half full?
Practice smiling at the world! 'If you smile at the world the world smiles back'. Cheer up a lonely old lady in the park, smile at the children in their buggies, smile at the dogs if you

can't muster their owners, smile at the sunshine on your face. Try a good belly laugh when you do your relaxation. It is a wonderful stress buster, no-one will hear you and if they do it is totally infectious!

Relaxation /Meditation/ Sleep.

A good thing to do regularly is relaxation. You can join a yoga class or meditation group, or try a self-help hypnosis tape. Practice at night when you can't sleep and it is quiet with no distractions. Another good time is after lunch, to give you a total break from the day. Give yourself no more than 20 minutes lying on your bed in the complete quiet. Turn off the phone, radio, TV etc.

Lie on your back on the bed, perhaps with a pillow under your knees for extra comfort, with just one pillow under your head. Place your hands gently across your lower abdomen or down beside you, palms up. If you are comfortable getting down and back up, you can also try lying on a rug on the warm floor, with a small cushion under your head and maybe under your knees.

Gently roll your head from side to side, easing out some of the neck tension, not forcing it or making it hurt.

Let go of the tension in your body. Do it bit by bit starting at the top of your head, working down. Clench and unclench your jaw and relax your face muscles. If you can't allow some bits of our body to relax, tense up the muscles of that area as you breathe in and then blow out your breath loudly between your lips [like blowing out a candle] while you relax your muscles. Do it several times on each set of muscles if necessary.

Once your body starts to feel heavy, concentrate on your breathing. You are aiming to make it as slow and deep as you comfortably can without straining or forcing anything. Counting in on 4 and out on 8 helps focus the mind.

The simplest form of 'meditation' is just being present and feeling your body heavy and relaxed all the way up and down. You can do visual journeys to nice places too, but these are easier if led by someone in a group. Whatever you decide to do, try to let your thoughts be easy and peaceful for a while. If your thoughts start to get anxious and busy, gently come back to the counting of the breath, as our thoughts can become like undisciplined monkeys, jumping from tree to tree!

You may drift off into a light sleep which can be very refreshing, but don't allow yourself more than a ten minute nap during the day or it disturbs your night sleeping. Relaxation can be a wonderful way of spending the wakeful hours of the night and may help you get back to sleep too.
Try if possible to be content with <u>not</u> sleeping! Taking sleeping tablets has very harmful effects long-term, especially on toxicity levels, and many of them are also addictive. One can survive with only a couple of hours sleep, providing the body is resting and gently relaxed.

The preparation for night sleep is also important. If your brain is busy with daytime thoughts, anxieties and stimulation it is buzzing by the time evening comes. Caffeine will not help either, so AVOID this completely.

Although you may have 'Fibrofog' most of the day and feel tired, muzzy and depressed, your brain just won't switch itself off! So try a simple routine of a warm relaxing bath [not too hot] with some Lavender essential oil in it about an hour before you settle. Lavender is a very good calming herb which can be used often; as lavender bags on the pillow, oil burners in the bedroom, bath essence, rub on sticks on the temples and even as herb tea.

Other calming herbs include valerian, which can be taken as drops in water, or as tea. Also hops can be drunk, homeopathic rye [Avena Sativa from Weleda] and chamomile. The latter is a diuretic, so although it is super if you feel stressed it is not so good at bedtime. Check out a good herbal book for exact recipes on how to make these, and you will become fascinated in the whole subject of how the plants around us can help us to stay healthy. Getting to know and love these plants, growing them yourself and feeling they are your friends is part of the healing process of becoming more grounded and at one with Mother Earth.

Oats are a very good tummy settler if you feel like a snack before bed. A bowl of fairly runny porridge with a little honey can send you off to sleep easily. Avoid adding sugar, which will wake you up again! Hot chocolate, ovaltine and other similar bedtime drinks all contain chemicals and high sugar and should be avoided.

An Indian recipe a friend gave me is very good to help you sleep. Put some Soya or rice milk in a pan. Add a couple of crushed cardamom pods, a cinnamon stick and a small teaspoon of turmeric. As an occasional treat you can also grate a little real chocolate block into it too. Simmer slowly for 5 minutes and strain. When cooled to blood temperature, add a half teaspoon of local honey [overheating honey kills all the helpful enzymes] and sip slowly. Yummy!

Avoid watching TV late into the evening. The flashing images on the screen strain the fine eye muscles as well as over stimulating your nerve pathways. Often we are producing Adrenaline as we watch exciting programmes but we do not use it to run, but it pumps around our bodies and creates acid in the system. TV has become so much part of our culture we have forgotten how damaging it can be to people with sensitive nervous systems [which YOU have!]

It is the same with any electronic equipment. Try to avoid the computer screen, completely if life allows it, but strictly limited if you have to be linked in to cyber space for your work; especially in the evenings or if you have a patch of not sleeping well. Turn things off at the plug if you can, rather than staying on standby.

Mobile or portable telephones also give off electromagnetic waves which over stimulate the nervous system. Avoid long telephone conversations, especially in the evening, unless you are using an old fashioned handset.

Listening to gentle music and having a short read in bed or writing a daily diary helps you slow down and drift off peacefully.

Avoid other 'props' such as a whisky or glass of wine to make you soporific, they only poison your system.

Massage is a super comfort for achy muscles. A very good rub across your shoulders and back or on your feet with Lavender oil can help you to sleep. If you do not have a partner, or he/she is unable to help, then a warm footbath followed by rubbing oil into your feet yourself can be a super pick-you up at any time of the day.

Try using Rosemary oil first thing in the morning. It is warming and stimulating to the circulation and uplifting to the Spirit.

Exercise.

Doctors and researchers are coming to the thought that exercise HELPS Fibromyalgia. If you take regular exercise they say you will loose weight, sleep better and be less stiff and achy. But how is this achieved when you feel achy all over, doing exercise seems to make you worse, and you have no energy for day to day living let alone exercising?

The key here is to listen to your body and do as much as regularly as possible.

Remember that taking in Oxygen is vital to life, so breathing well during the day is another key to success. Many people, especially who have been stressed long-term, will have poor breathing, using only the upper part of the chest, so practise taking a deep breath when you remember [but never force it or over breathe], and going out into fresh air is vital every day.

Start by having a very short walk outside 2-3 times a day. Never miss your daily walk, however small. Even if you can only stagger to the garden gate and back, never miss it. If you have to drive to the shops then park up somewhere nice on the way there or back and take a ten minute walk. Gradually increase the speed. Some days you will hurt all over and will crawl along, but keep breathing and enjoy the sun or rain on your face and look around at the trees and flowers, the running dogs and children. They are full of life energy and you can absorb it from them.

Don't attempt to go to the gym and pound on the treadmill for an hour. You will feel ghastly for several days afterwards! Instead take a slightly longer walk firstly on the flat, and as you get fitter up a slope. Don't attempt pushing yourself up big hills too soon, you will regret it afterwards. Give yourself little goals to go a bit further every day.

Swimming is wonderfully relaxing and gives your muscles the chance of a gentle workout, but again build up gradually and beware that you may be sensitive to the strong chemicals in some swimming pools. Shower well afterwards and drink plenty of good water.

Try using a bicycle, on the flat first and gradually increase to small hills. Electric bicycles are now becoming popular to help you up the hills.

Muscles **deteriorate after 6 hours** of not being used, so the key to getting fit is a little and often gradually increasing and not missing two or three days.

You will be able to do less in the winter cold, when a low pressure is coming over, or if you haven't slept well. If you feel acidic because you have overdone things, just be loving with yourself and start your fitness programme again from a low level. Don't ever give up exercising as you will 'lose it if you don't use it!'

The main thing with exercise is enjoying it. Feel at one with your body and don't push yourself. It will enliven your circulation and help you detoxify.

Avoid the trap of thinking you are going to end up in a wheelchair, or need a mobility scooter. We all age and dehydration will effect our joints and muscles more as we age, but if you keep well hydrated and eat the right food you will not age any faster, either physically or mentally, than the average healthy person. We Fibros have a label of sickness, but we can live a healthy life despite it!

Weight loss/ gain.

Most people with Fibromyalgia are overweight. The reason for this is not necessarily eating too many calories, so the answer is NOT to go to a slimming club, [although being weighed every week may encourage you in other ways.] The reason is that our bodies store excess acid in the body as fat. This is actually a fantastic mechanism which avoids the acid damaging the vital organs, and as soon as you start to become less acidic you may notice a natural weight loss. Fats only break down gradually though, so don't expect super miracles. A healthy body is naturally the right weight. You will also be eating the right sort of foods, avoiding sugars and wrong fats and increasing exercise, so weight loss will be a bonus. Being overweight is not good for anyone and can also be one of the CAUSES of Fibromyalgia. Which comes first; the chicken or the egg? If you are underweight you may also find you start putting on a bit with your new health regime.

Rhythm and self discipline.

The body has natural rhythms over 24 hours and also the cycles of the seasons affect us profoundly. The body craves to be in the natural cycle of the earth and heavens, as we are a tiny part of the whole moving universe.

Planets and far away stars can affect us as much as the moon cycles and the happenings on this earth, including manmade things like wars and pollution.

When things are out of harmony, as they are in many places on this earth at the present time, our bodies find it harder to maintain a natural rhythm which is vital for health.

It is ever more important therefore if one is ill or 'dis-eased' to try and recreate the rhythm which the body craves. Simple things such as going to bed at the same time [and not too late], eating at the same time of day, taking exercise and activity at the same time, all helps towards stabilising what has become an out-of-balance organism. All these things require self discipline, which will strengthen as you become healthier.

We all have our natural rhythms and are unique because we all chose to be born at a different moment in time when the universal bodies were in a particular relationship to each other. Some chose to be born with the Zodiac sign Libra on the horizon, while others chose Virgo. Some have their sun in Aries, others in Aquarius etc. Some have the Moon in Leo, others in Capricorn. Astrology is a highly complex subject, but if studied seriously can be helpful in shedding light on our imbalances and enabling us to understand some of our dis-ease. We can then accept more easily the struggles of our present life and know that it is all part of the great pattern of the Universal Energy. A professional astrological consultation may be helpful to you at some point on your journey.

Conclusion

By this stage of reading you may be feeling quite angry or confused by the positive [or unrealistic?] attitude which I am putting across. The glass can be half empty or half full in any situation. Everyone is different, but we are all born with the potential for leading the sort of life which will give us our 'soul lessons.' What we do with our potential is our unique journey through life. If we have <u>abused</u> our bodies beyond their natural inherited limits [which most people with Fibromyalgia have done in earlier years] then our lesson is to come into a state of balance again and care for ourselves in a new and more conscious way. It can be a very revealing path to work with and if we can take it on joyfully and accept the idiosyncrasies of our bodies we are already on the path of recovery. Our emotions and mental responses to these challenges are part of this journey. Any 'Disability' is a life challenge and Fibromyalgia can be our own personal challenge as well as that of our family. Other peoples' attitudes to Fibromyalgia can be formed by our own attitude, while we learn to live in a more healthy and harmonious way, which is exactly what this condition can help us to achieve.

I hope very much that you have found something in this 'Toolkit' which may be of use to you and that maybe you can pass some tips on to others suffering from Fibromyalgia.

In Sidmouth, East Devon, our support group meets the first Friday of each month at Twyford House, Coburg Road, from 10a.m.

Angela Bea, March 2012

Appendix 1.

Notes;

This list of Alkaline and Acid foods was compiled from material found in Dr Robert Young's 'The pH Miracle' book and is not definitive. All foods can be listed as either acid [-] or alkaline [+] depending on the effect they have on the body and the rate of metabolism.

As can be seen from the list, most first class proteins are highly acid as are also sugars and junk foods. It is therefore important to try and eat as many alkaline foods [vegetables] as possible and limit the amount of acid foods. Fruit is acid too, because it contains a lot of sugar.

A very helpful in depth book on acid/alkaline balance is by Christopher Vasey. [The Acid- Alkaline diet for optimum Health].
He describes in detail the chemistry of metabolism and shows also how some people cannot cope with 'weak acids', which includes acid or sweet fruits, yoghourt and acid cheeses, honey and vinegar. Check it out if the normal pH diet isn't working for you. He also gives in depth details on testing for acidity in the body.

PH testing sticks for urine and saliva are available on-line and are the only accurate way of testing whether you are acid or alkaline. The urine normally tests acid first thing in the morning, but thereafter should ideally read between 7 and 7.5.

A useful rule of thumb for a maintenance diet would be 20% acid food and 80% alkaline, but this depends on the individual and their acid level at any one time.

Note; the unusual grasses listed are ingredients of the 'Supergreens' produced by the company 'Innerlight' [www.innerlightinc.com].This powder can be mixed with water and drunk throughout the day. It is available on-line. Several other companies now produce green powders made from wheat grass and other grasses and alkalising foods. It is worth doing your own research.

www.Energiseforlife.com is a very useful English website with lots of aspects of this complex subject covered; diet, water, alkaline mineral drops, supplements and lots of support.

I have been unable to confirm the acidity/alkalinity of Quinoa, barley, and oats. Note that rice becomes neutral if soaked for some hours before cooking. All sprouted foods become more alkaline.

Olive oil is alkaline, whereas Sunflower oil and margarine are acid. Avoid marg with hydrogenated fats.

The pH of water is dependent on the source. Ionisers can be adjusted to create quite alkaline water [pH 10] and when a sufficient volume of this is drunk it helps the whole system.

Becoming more alkaline, you will loose weight, get more energy and boost your immune system.

Pathological Cells, such as cancer cells, HIV, Candida and bacteria/microbes in the blood revert back to healthy cells when bathed in an alkaline solution. This is important biochemical research which Dr Young has done.

Because of this important work one can assume that anyone suffering 'dis-ease' is in fact running acid. Dehydration is another huge cause of acidity.

Remember that everyone's body is unique and what works for one person may not be right for another!

The pH of some foods.

Vegetables

Peas +0.5
Asparagus +1.1
Artichokes +1.3
Comfrey +1.5
Green cabbage March +2.0
Potatoes +2.0
Lettuce +2.2
Onion +3.0
Cauliflower +3.1
White radish +3.1
Swede +3.1
White cabbage +3.3
Green cabbage December +4.0
Savoy +4.5
Lamb's lettuce +4.8
New peas +5.1
Kohlrabi +5.1
Courgette +5.7
Red cabbage +6.3
Rhubarb +6.3
Horseradish +6.8
Leeks +7.2
Watercress +7.7
Spinach March +8.0
Turnip +8.0
Lime +8.2
Chives +8.3
Carrot +9.5
Lemon +9.9
French beans +11.2
Fresh beetroot +11,3
Spinach not March +13.1

Garlic +13.2
Celery +13.3
Tomato +13.6
Cabbage lettuce +14.1
Endive +14.1
Sorrel +11.2
Avocado +15.6
Red radish +16.7
Cayenne +18.8
Straw grass +21.4
Horsetail +21.7
Dog Grass + 22.6
Dandelion +22.7
Barley Grass +28.7
Soy Sprouts +29.5
Sprouted radish +28.4
Alfalfa Grass +29.3
Cucumber +31.5
Wheat Grass +33.8
Black Radish +39.4

Organic grain and legumes
Brown rice -12.5
Wheat -10.1
Oats? acid?
Barley? Acid?
Brown rice soaked 24 hours neutral.
Quinoa ? +
Buckwheat -0.5
Millet -0.5
Lentils +0.6
Soy flour +2.5
Tofu +3.2
Lima beans +12
Cooked soy +12.8
Soy nuts +26.5
Soy lecithin +38.0
Sprouted = more alkaline.

Nuts and seeds
Pistachios -16.6
Peanuts -12.8
Cashews -9.3
Wheat germ -11.4
Walnuts -8.0
Pumpkin seeds -5.4
Sunflower seeds -5.4
Macadamia nuts -3.2
Hazel nuts -2.0
Flax seeds -1.3
Brazil nuts -0.5
Sesame seeds +0.5
Cumin seeds +1.1
Fennel seeds + 1.3
Caraway seeds +2.3
Almonds +3.6

Fats
Margarine -7.6
Sunflower oil -6.4
Butter -3.9
Ghee -1.6
Coconut milk -1.5
Olive oil +1.0
Borage oil +3.2
Flax seed oil +3.5
Evening primrose oil +4.1
Marine lipids +4.7

Fish and meat

Freshwater fish -11.8
Ocean fish -20.1
Oysters -5.0
Pork -38.0
Veal -35.0
Beef -34.5
Chicken -20.0
Eggs -20.0
Liver -3.0
Organ meats -3.0

Milk etc.
Hard cheese -18.1
Quark -17.3
Cream -3.9
Buttermilk +1.3

Bread
White bread -10.0
Biscuits -6.5
Wholemeal bread -6.5
Rye bread -2.5

Sweets

Sweeteners -26.5
White sugar -17.6
Beet sugar -15.1
Molasses -14.6
Fructose -9.5
Milk sugar -9.5
Barley malt syrup -9.3
Brown rice syrup -8.7
Honey -7.6

Condiments

Vinegar -39.4
Soy sauce -36.2
Mustard -19.2
Mayonnaise -12.5
Ketchup -12.4

Drinks

Spirits -28.6 _ -38.7
Sweetened fruit juice -33.4
Tea -27.1
Beer -26.8
Coffee -25.1
Wine -16.4
Fruit juice natural -8.7
Mineral-water –
acid, depending on brand
Tap water - acid
Alkalized water -+

Appendix 2. Useful books, references and websites.

This list is by no means conclusive and many more references may be found by buying one or two of these books, or browsing online. The journey has begun!

Websites;
- ukfibromyalgia.com [Online forums, support, articles]

- rightdiagnosis.com [Define your symptoms]

- nationalpainfoundation.org [self-management strategies]

Books;
- The pH Miracle. Dr R. Young [Time Warner pub.]

- Cellular Awakening. Barbara Wren [www.hayhouse.co.uk]

- The Healing journey. Matthew Manning [www.piatkus.co.uk]

- Chronic Fatigue, ME, and Fibromyalgia. The Natural Recovery Plan. Alison Adams [www.watkinspublishing.co.uk]

- Fibromyalgia Naturally. Patti Chandler

- Fibromyalgia Basics. Patti Chandler.

- The Acid-Alkaline Diet. Christopher Vasey. [Healing Arts Press]

- The Fibromyalgia Healing Diet [includes yeast and sugars]. Christine Craggs-Hinton. [Sheldon Press]

- Candida Albicans. Shirley Trickett. [www.Thorsons.com]

- Cooking without. Barbara Cousins [Thorsons]

- The Alkaline Diet Recipe Book. Ross Bridgeford. [www.Energiseforlife.com]

Printed in Great Britain
by Amazon.co.uk, Ltd.,
Marston Gate.